MyWW

New Complete

Cookbook 2024

Increase Your Energy and Get Young Again with
Simple and Flavorful WW Freestyle Recipes

By
Dr. Blanche Fleming

Table of Contents

Bacon and Goat Cheese Salad Recipe
Prep Time: 25 Minutes, Cook Time: 15 Minutes,
SERVINGS :6, Points Value: 6

INGREDIENTS:

- ➤ 1 1/2 servings Atkins Low Carb Wheat Bread , 6 medium slice (yield after cooking) Bacon & 4 cups shredded Cos or Romaine Lettuce

- ➤ 2 cups chopped Endive, 3 tablespoons chopped Chives & 8 ounces Goat Cheese (Soft)

- ➤ 1 large Egg (Whole), 2 tablespoons Extra Virgin Olive Oil & 1 1/2 tablespoons Red Wine Vinegar

- ➤ 1 tablespoon Dijon Mustard & 3/4 teaspoon Black Pepper

DIRECTIONS:

- ▪ At first Use the Atkins recipe to make Atkins Low Carb Wheat Bread, you will need 1 1/2 slices, toast the slices then blend in a blender into fine crumbs in step 3.

FOR SALAD:

- ▪ Next Cook bacon in a large nonstick skillet over medium heat, turning once, until crisp, about 6 to 7 minutes. Transfer with a slotted spoon to paper towels.

- ▪ Then Reserve 1 tablespoon of bacon drippings.

- ▪ After that Chop the Romaine lettuce, endive and chives then combine in a serving bowl and set aside.

- ▪ Menahwhile In a food processor or blender, process bread to make crumbs; spread crumbs on a plate.

- ▪ Later Place goat cheese slices cut side down on work surface and press lightly to flatten. In a small bowl whisk the egg and dip each slice of cheese allowing the excess to drip off. Place on crumbs, pressing to coat evenly and completely.

- Meanwhile Wipe out bacon skillet with a paper towel; add oil and heat over medium heat. Add goat-cheese patties and cook until browned, about 2 minutes per side (reduce heat if browning occurs too fast or cheese is melting).

- In the mentime Transfer to a plate lined with paper towels.

- Moreover Remove skillet from heat but reserve the bacon grease fro the dressing.

DRESSING:

- In the next step Add reserved bacon drippings, olive oil, vinegar, mustard and pepper to skillet. Whisk to combine. Add warm dressing and bacon to bowl with greens. Toss to combine.

- Finally Arrange salad on individual serving plates and top each with a goat-cheese patty.

Nutriotional Info:

13.8g Protein, 17.4g Fat, 1.5g Fiber, 221.7 Calories

Grilled Asian Eggplant with Miso and Sesame Oil Recipe

Prep Time: 10 Minutes, Cook Time: 5 Minutes,
SERVINGS : 4, Points Value: 5

INGREDIENTS:

- ➢ 1/8 serving Hoisin Sauce, 1 1/3 tablespoons Toasted Sesame Oil & 1 teaspoon Garlic

- ➢ 1/3 tablespoon chopped Shallots

- ➢ 1 tablespoon Organic Tamari, 2/3 tablespoon Miso Paste, all styles & 2 tablespoons Canola Oil

- ➢ 16 ounces Eggplant, 50 leaves Basil & 2 ounces Dry Roasted Peanuts (with Salt)

DIRECTIONS:

- ▪ Miso paste can be made from barley, rice or soy.

- ▪ This recipe calls for the soy kind, brown is more mellow tasting than red or white.

- ▪ Asian eggplants are narrow and straight, with a sweeter taste than the larger, rounder Italian ones.

- ▪ Holy basil is best for this recipe because it has an anise flavor.

- ▪ Substitute another sweet basil if you cannot find it. If you don't have a grill, use the broiler instead.

- ▪ At the starting period Prepare the topping in a small bowl, thoroughly mixing the Hoisin sauce, 1 teaspoon toasted sesame oil, minced garlic, chopped shallot, tamari and miso paste. Set aside.

- Next Prepare the marinade by mixing together the remaining 1 tablespoon of toasted sesame and canola oil.

- Then Brush on the eggplant and let stand for 30 minutes or up to an hour.

- Meanwhil ePreheat the grill to medium. Grill eggplant halves, skin side down, for 2-3 minutes. Turn and grill for another 2-3 minutes on the other side.

- Later Using a butter knife, spread the topping on the cut side of the eggplant halves.

- Moreover Sprinkle with basil and 1/4 roasted chopped peanuts (if using) before serving. Enjoy!

- Steel's Rocky Mountain Hoisin Sauce contains no sugar. To chiffonade is to cut into narrow strips. Stack the basil leaves, roll them tightly and then slice into thin strips with a sharp knife.

- Finally when the dish is ready to serve, serve it and enjoy!!!

Nutriotional Info:

5.7g Protein, 19.2g Fat, 5.2g Fiber, 223 Calories

Sweet Potato and Spinach Salad Recipe

Prep Time: 10 Minutes, Cook Time: 8 Minutes,
SERVINGS : 4, Points Value: 1

INGREDIENTS:

- ➤ 1/2 small Red Onion, 1 tablespoon Extra Virgin Olive Oil & 1/2 fluid ounce Freshly Squeezed Orange Juice

- ➤ 1/2 tablespoon Sodium and Sugar Free Rice Vinegar & 3/4 teaspoon Salt

- ➤ 1/4 teaspoon Black Pepper, 1 sweetpotato, 5" long Sweet Potato

- ➤ 4 cups Baby Spinach & 1 small Sweet Red Pepper

DIRECTIONS:

- At first Combine onion, oil, juice, vinegar, salt, and pepper in a bowl.

- Next Cut potato into 1/2-inch dice. Put potato dice in a small saucepan with enough lightly salted water to cover and bring to a boil.

- Then Cook until tender but not mushy, about 8 minutes. Drain in a colander.

- After thatIn a large bowl, toss potato, spinach and pepper with dressing.

- Finally Serve immediately.

Nutriotional Info:

1.5g Protein, 3.5g Fat, 2.2g Fiber, 75cal Calories

Keto Lettuce-Wrapped Chicken Burger with Avocado and Tomato Recipe

Prep Time: 5 Minutes, Cook Time: 12 Minutes,
SERVINGS: 6, Points Value: 9

INGREDIENTS:

- ➢ 42 ounces Ground Chicken, 3 each California Avocados & 3 large whole (3" diameter) Red Tomatoes

- ➢ 18 leaves Butterhead Lettuce (Includes Boston and Bibb Types)

DIRECTIONS:

- ▪ At first Form ground chicken into a patty and season with salt and freshly ground black pepper.

- ▪ Next Grill or fry in a non-stick pan (with 1 tsp of oil or oil spray) until it is nicely browned and no longer pink in the center.

- ▪ Then Top with sliced avocado and tomato then wrap in lettuce leaves.

- ▪ Finally when the dish is ready to serve, serve it and enjoy!!!

Nutriotional Info:

31.2g Protein, 27.7g Fat, 7.2g Fiber, 412.6 Calories

Spicy Turkey Club Recipe

INGREDIENTS:

- ➤ 12 servings Atkins Low Carb Wheat Bread , 3 tablespoons chopped Scallions or Spring Onions & 3 teaspoons Sriracha Hot Chili Sauce

- ➤ 1 tablespoon Fresh Lime Juice, 1 pound Turkey Breast Meat (Fryer-Roasters, Cooked, Roasted) & 1/2 teaspoon Garlic

- ➤ 8 leaves Radicchio, 1 small whole (2-2/5" diameter) Red Tomato

- ➤ 8 medium slice (yield after cooking) Bacon & 1/2 cup Real Mayonnaise

DIRECTIONS:

- ▪ At first Cook bacon, set aside on a paper towel to cool.

- ▪ While bacon is cooking, combine mayonnaise, scallions, lime juice, chili sauce (to taste), minced garlic, salt and pepper to taste in a small bowl.

- ▪ Next To assemble: Spread bread slices with mayonnaise.

- ▪ Then Lay 2-3 turkey slices on top of 4 bread slices and top with radicchio leaf, tomato slice and bacon.

- ▪ After that Repeat layering once and then cover with the last 4 slices of bread.

- Meanwhile Insert toothpicks to hold sandwiches in place before slicing.

- Finally Serve immediately.

Nutriotinal Info:

38.9g Fat, 3.6g Fiber, 637.3 Calories

Vanilla Coffee Frappé Recipe

INGREDIENTS:

- ➢ 2 cup ice cubes Tap Water & 1 each Atkins Creamy Vanilla Shake

- ➢ 3 teaspoon, dries Instant Coffee (Dry Powder) & 3 tablespoons Heavy Cream

DIRECTIONS:

- ▪ At first Combine 2 cups of ice in a blender with Atkins Creamy Vanilla Shake, heavy cream and instant coffee.

- ▪ Next Blend until thoroughly combined and all the ice is crushed.

- ▪ Finally Serve with a dollop of whipped cream if desired. Also terrific with 1/2 tsp ground cinnamon.

Nutriotional Info:

16.2g Protein, 25.6g Fat , 5g Fiber, 320.7 Calories

Keto Shrimp with Avocado and Tomato Salad Recipe

Prep Time: 5 Minutes, Cook Time: 5 Minutes

SERVING :6 , Points Value: 4

INGREDIENTS:

- ➢ 1 serving Keto Creamy Italian Dressing & 12 large Shrimps

- ➢ 1/2 fruit without skin and seed California Avocados & 5 Cherry Tomatoes

- ➢ 1 sprig Cilantro & 2 cups Romaine, raw, hearts

DIRECTIONS:

- At first Use the Atkins recipe to make Creamy Italian Dressing, you will need 2 tablespoons.

- Next Steam shrimp in a steamer basket over boiling water until they turn pink and just start to curl.

- Then Immediately transfer to a bowl filled with ice and cold water.

- After that Drain , pat dry, peel and devein. Or use frozen precooked shrimp that have been thoroughly thawed. Coarsely chop if large and put into a bowl.

- Meanwhile Add the chopped avocado, halved cherry tomatoes, chopped cilantro and Romaine in the bowl with the shrimp and toss with the dressing.

- Finally Serve immediately.

Nutriotional Info:

Protein 23.7g, Fat , 8g Fiber ,354.6 Calories

Chard and Cheese Casserole Recipe

Prep Time: 20 Minutes, Cook Time: 55 Minutes,
SERVINGS: 6, Points Value: 5

INGREDIENTS:

- ➢ 2 tablespoons Extra Virgin Olive Oil, 3/4 pound Swiss Chard & 1 medium (approx 2-3/4" long, 2-1/2" diameter) Sweet Red Peppers

- ➢ 1 small Onion, 1/2 teaspoon Salt & 1/4 teaspoon Black Pepper

- ➢ 1 1/2 cups shredded Muenster Cheese & 1/2 cup Parmesan Cheese (Grated)

DIRECTIONS

- At first Heat oven to 350°F. Grease an 8x8-inch baking dish.

- Next Prepare the chard by folding each leaf in half and cutting out the hard stem/vein.

- Then Roll up the leafs and coarsely chop them then dice the stems keeping each separate.

- Meanwhile Heat 1 tablespoon oil in a large Dutch oven or heavy pot over high heat.

- After that Add the chard leaves to the pot and cook 3 - 4 minutes, until wilted.

- In the meantime Drain in colander; press with the back of a spoon to extract excess liquid discard liquid and set aside.

- In the next step Heat remaining tablespoon of oil in a large skillet over medium heat.

- Later Dice the bell pepper and white onion. Place in the pan with the diced chard stems and sauté for 8 minutes, until softened.

- Moreover Mix in chard leaves; toss to coat. Season with salt and pepper.

- Mix in Muenster cheese & Spoon into prepared baking dish. E

- venly sprinkle Parmesan cheese over top. Cover with aluminum foil; bake 30 minutes.

- Finally Uncover and cook 10 minutes more, until cheese is brown and bubbl & when the dish is ready to serve, serve it and enjoy!!!

Nutriotional Info:

11.2g Protein, 15.6g Fat, 1.5g Fiber, 200.7 Calories

Radicchio, Gorgonzola and Bacon Salad Recipe

Prep Time: 5 Minutes, Cook Time: 15 Minutes,
SERVINGS : 4, Points Value: 5

INGREDIENTS:

- ➢ 2 medium slice (yield after cooking) Bacon & 3 tablespoons Extra Virgin Olive Oil

- ➢ 1 tablespoon Fresh Lemon Juice & 1 head (5" dia) Butterhead Lettuce (Includes Boston and Bibb Types)

- ➢ 1/2 pound Radicchio, 2 ounces Gorgonzola Cheese & 2 tablespoons Parsley

DIRECTIONS:

- At first Cook bacon until crisp; transfer to a paper towel to drain. & Crumble bacon; set aside.

- Next In a large bowl whisk together olive oil, lemon juice, and salt and pepper to taste.

- Then Add gently torn Boston lettuce, radicchio, cheese and parsley.

- After that Toss gently to coat. Transfer to plates; sprinkle with bacon.

- Finally when the dish is ready to serve,serve it and enjoy!!!!

Nutriotional Info:

5.9g Protein, 16.1g Fat, 1g Fiber, 181.2 Calories

String Bean and Snow Pea Salad

INGREDIENTS:

- ➤ 5 1/4 ounces Snowpeas (Pea Pod), 1/3 pound Green Snap Beans & 2 tablespoons Extra Virgin Olive Oil

- ➤ 1 tablespoon White Wine Vinegar & 1/2 teaspoon Salt

- ➤ 1/2 teaspoon Sucralose Based Sweetener (Sugar Substitute) & 1/2 teaspoon leaf Tarragon

DIRECTIONS:

- At first Steam string beans in a steamer basket in a medium pot over boiling lightly salted water 3-4 minutes until crisp-tender.

- Next Add snow peas during the last minute of cooking time.

- Then Drain and place in serving dish. Add oil, vinegar, salt, sugar substitute and tarragon.

- Finally Toss to coat vegetables evenly and serve warm. Or refrigerate for at least 1 hour and serve chilled.

Nutriotional INfo:

1.7g Protein, 6.9g Fat, 2.2g Fiber, 87.7 Calories

Keto Salmon Fillets with Dill Mousseline Recipe

Prep Time: 20 Minutes, Cook Time: 5 Minutes,

SERVINGS : 4, Points Value: 12

INGREDIENTS:

- ➤ 1/3 cup Heavy Cream, 24 ounces boneless, raw Salmon & 1/2 fruit (2-3/8" diameter) Lemon

- ➤ 1 teaspoon Salt, 1/2 teaspoon Black Pepper & 1/8 cup sprig Dill

- ➤ 1 tablespoon Parsley, 2 tablespoons chopped Onions & 2 large Egg Yolks

- ➤ 1 tablespoon Fresh Lemon Juice & 5 tablespoons Unsalted Butter Stick

DIRECTIONS:

- At first Heat oven to 375°F & Whip cream with a whisk or electric beater until soft peaks form; set aside. Line a baking pan with aluminum foil.

- Next Season salmon with juice from lemon, salt, and pepper.

- Then Mix 1 tablespoon dill, minced parsley, and small diced white onion in a small bowl.

- After that Heat a large nonstick skillet over high heat for 2 minutes.

- Meaanwhile Sear salmon on both sides 2 minutes per side until nicely browned & Transfer to baking pan.

- In the meantime Pat herb mixture onto salmon & Bake 5 to 6 minutes for medium doneness.

- Later Remove from oven, transfer to warmed plates.

- While salmon is baking, prepare Hollandaise sauce: Place egg yolks, lemon juice, in a food processor or blender and process briefly.

- With the motor running, pour in melted butter in a very thin stream.

- Sauce should thicken slowly & Season to taste with salt and pepper.

- Before the final step Gently fold Hollandaise sauce and remaining dill into whipped cream.

- Finally Spoon sauce over fish, serve it and enjoy

Nutriotional Info:

38.9g Protein, 34.1g Fat, 0.5g Fiber, 478 Calories

Pepper Jack Quesadillas Recipe

Prep Time: 15 Minutes, Cook Time: 28 Minutes, SERVINGS :6, Points Value: 3

INGREDIENTS:

- ➤ 2 tablespoons Canola Vegetable Oil, 1/2 teaspoon Salt & 3/4 cup shredded Monterey Jack Cheese

- ➤ 1/2 ounce Cilantro (Coriander), 2 medium (2-1/2" diameter) Onions & 6 tortillas Low Carb Tortillas

DIRECTIONS:

- At first Heat oil in a large nonstick skillet over medium-high heat & Add diced onion and salt; cook, stirring occasionally, until golden, 10 to 12 minutes.

- Next Transfer onions to a small bowl and cool. Wipe out skillet & Place tortillas on work surface.

- Then Sprinkle the lower half of each with 1/4 cup cheese, 1 tablespoon white onion and 1/2 teaspoon cilantro.

- After that Fold each tortilla in half over filling to form a semicircle & Heat the skillet over medium heat.

- In the meantime Add the quesadillas two or three at a time, and cook until lightly browned and the cheese has melted, about 3 to 4 minutes per side.

- Finally Transfer the quesadillas to a cutting board, and repeat with remaining ingredients & Cut quesadillas into four wedges.

Nutriotional Info:

6.6g Protein, 9g Fat, 3.4g Fiber, 127.4 Calories

Fried Hazelnut-Crusted Calamari with Spicy Tomato Sauce Recipe

Prep Time: 10 Minutes, Cook Time: 15 Minutes,
SERVINGS : 6, Points Value: 10

INGREDIENTS:

- ➢ 2/3 serving Atkins Soy-Free Flour Mix, 1 tablespoon Extra Virgin Olive Oil & 1 tablespoon Parsley

- ➢ 1/4 teaspoon Crushed Red Pepper Flakes,1 1/3 cups Tomato Sauce (Canned) & 1 cup chopped Hazelnuts or Filberts

- ➢ 1/4 teaspoon dried cayenne chili pepper, ground, 1 pound Squid (Mixed Species) & 1/4 cup Peanut Oil

- ➢ 1/8 teaspoon Salt & 1 fruit (2-1/8" diameter) Lemon

DIRECTIONS:

- Use the Atkins recipe to make Atkins Soy-Free Flour Mix, you will need 2/3 cup & Use 2 cups refined peanut oil for frying in this recipe.

- For sauce: Next In a large skillet, heat olive oil over medium heat.

- Then Add parsley and red pepper flakes and sauté for 1 minute.

- After that Add tomato sauce and bring to a simmer. Cook, stirring occasionally, for 5 minutes (sauce may be made up to two days in advance).

- Meanwhile In a food processor, process hazelnuts, flour mix and cayenne until nuts are finely ground, about 1 minute.

- In the next step Transfer to a shallow bowl. Dredge calamari in mixture, tapping to remove any excess, and set aside.

- After a while Heat oil in a deep sauce pot until temperature reaches 375°F.

- Later Fry calamari in batches, 30 seconds per batch, until firm and light golden.

- Finally Transfer to a paper-towel-lined plate to drain & Sprinkle with salt and serve with sauce and lemon wedges.

Nutriotional Info:

28.5g Protein, 32.5g Fat , 5.8g Fiber, 461.2Calories

Keto Mustard-Cream Sauce Recipe

Prep Time: 5 Minutes, Cook Time: 0 Minutes,

SERVINGS :6, Points Value: 4

INGREDIENTS:

- ➢ 2/3 cup Heavy Cream, liquid & 1 small (3" long) Scallions or Spring Onions
- ➢ 1 1/2 tablespoons Original Stone Ground Mustard, 1/4 teaspoon Black Pepper & 1/8 teaspoon Salt

DIRECTIONS:

- At first Serve this savory sauce over chicken, pork or veal cutlets, or poached salmon or chicken breasts & Each serving is 2 Tbsp.

- Next Pour cream into a small skillet and bring to a boil over high heat.

- Then Reduce heat to medium high, stir in diced scallion and cook, stirring frequently, until cream thickens slightly, about 3 minutes.

- Later Remove from heat and stir in mustard, pepper and salt.

- Finally Taste and add salt if desired. Use immediately.

Nutriotional Info:

0.9g Protein, 15.2g Fat, 0.6g Fiber, 148.7 Calories

Turkey Ratatouille Recipe

INGREDIENTS:

- ➢ 24 oz, boneless, raw, without skin (yield after cooking) Turkey Cutlet & 4 tablespoons Extra Virgin Olive Oil

- ➢ 1 eggplant, unpeeled (approx 1-1/4 lb) Eggplant & 1 medium Zucchini

- ➢ 1 medium (approx 2-3/4" long, 2-1/2" diameter) Sweet Red Peppers & 1 cup Mushroom Pieces and Stems

- ➢ 1 teaspoon Garlic & 1/2 cup Tomato Puree (Without Salt Added, Canned)

- ➢ 1 teaspoon leaf Basil (Dried), 1/2 teaspoon Sucralose Based Sweetener (Sugar Substitute)

- ➢ 1/8 teaspoon Salt & 1/8 teaspoon Black Pepper

DIRECTIONS:

- ▪ At first Heat 1 tablespoon oil in a large skillet over medium heat.

- ▪ Next Sprinkle cutlets with salt and freshly ground black pepper.

- ▪ Then Sauté cutlets 3 minutes per side, just until lightly golden and cooked through. Transfer to a plate.

- ▪ Meanwhile Heat remaining oil in skillet. Add eggplant, zucchini and red pepper.

- ▪ In the meantime Sauté 5 minutes, stirring occasionally. Add mushrooms, garlic, tomato purée, basil and sugar substitute.

- Later Mix well; bring to a boil. Cover, reduce heat to low and simmer 5 minutes.

- Add salt and pepper.

- Return turkey and accumulated juices to skillet. Cook, uncovered 2-3 minutes, just until turkey is heated through.

- Finally Serve immediately.

Nutriotional Info:

42.7g Protein, 18.3g Fat, 6.7g Fiber, 391.3 Calories

Shrimp, Bacon and Avocado Salad Recipe

INGREDIENTS:

- ➤ 1 serving Keto Hot Bacon Vinaigrette & 12 medium Shrimp, raws

- ➤ 2 medium slice (yield after cooking) Bacon & 1/2 cup Jicama

- ➤ 1/2 fruit without skin and seed California Avocados & 2 cup, shredded or choppeds Mixed Salad Greens

DIRECTIONS:

- At first Use the Atkins recipe and reserve bacon drippings to make the Hot Bacon Vinaigrette, you will need 2 tablespoons.

- Next Place shrimp in steamer and steam until shrimp turn pink and curl up & This should take about 5 minutes once the water is boiling.

- Then Cook bacon slices on frying pan until crispy.

- After that Reserve drippings and make vinaigrette & Cut bacon into bits.

- Finally Toss cooked shrimp, bacon bits, diced jicama, diced avocado and greens with the dressing.

Nutriotional Info:

24.5g Protein, 38.3g Fat, 11.3g Fiber, 502.1 Calories

Keto Indian Tikka Chicken Recipe

Prep Time: 240 Minutes, Cook Time: 30 Minutes,
SERVINGS :4, Points Value: 6

INGREDIENTS:

- ➢ 1 cup Greek Yogurt - Plain (Container), 1/2 ounce Ginger & 1/2 ounce Cilantro (Coriander)

- ➢ 2 teaspoons Chili Powder, 1 tablespoon Peppermint, fresh & 24 ounce raw (yield after cooking, bone removed) Chicken Breast

- ➢ 1 tablespoon Extra Virgin Olive Oil, 1/2 teaspoon Salt & 1/4 teaspoon Black Pepper

DIRECTIONS:

- At first In shallow bowl combine yogurt, minced ginger, chopped cilantro, chili powder, coriander and 1 tsp freshly chopped mint and mix well.

- Next Add chicken, cover, and marinate refrigerated for between 4 hours and overnight.

- About 1 hour before cooking, remove chicken from refrigerator and bring to room temperature.

- Then Soak 4-6 thin wooden or bamboo skewers in water.

- After that Heat oven to 375°F. Thread chicken on skewers, place on a baking sheet and drizzle with oil.

- Meanwhile Sprinkle with salt. Bake 30 minutes, turning once halfway through cooking time, until golden brown and cooked through.

- Finally Sprinkle with chopped cilantro and garnish with the extra mint and a squeeze of lime (optional)

Nutriotional Info:

32.6g Protein, 10.6g Fat, 0.7g Fiber, 243.9 Calories

Keto Cornish Game Hens with Peach-Lime Glaze Recipe

Prep Time: 60 Minutes, Cook Time: 30 Minutes, SERVINGS : 6, Points Value: 3

INGREDIENTS:

- ➤ 3 bird wholes Chicken Meat (Cornish Game Hens) & 1 teaspoon Lime Zest

- ➤ 1/3 cup Lime Juice, 8 tablespoons Sugar Free Apricot Preserves

- ➤ 3 tablespoons Soy Sauce Tamari & 2 teaspoons Garlic

DIRECTIONS:

- At first Season hens with salt and pepper to taste; set aside & Zest and juice the lime.

- Next In a large bowl, mix jam, juice, soy sauce, minced garlic and 1 tsp zest.

- Then Add hens; toss to coat. Marinate 1 hour, turning occasionally.

- After that Prepare a medium grill. Remove hens from glaze; reserve glaze.

- In the meantime Place hens skin side down on greased grill grate, not directly over heat.

- Later Cover and cook 25 minutes, until no longer pink inside and juices run clear.

- Meanwhile, heat reserved glaze in a small saucepan over high heat; boil for 1 full minute.

- During last 5 minutes of cooking time, brush hens with glaze and cook directly over heat source for a crispy skin.

- Finally Serve with remaining glaze.

Nutriotional Info:

25.1g Protein, 4g Fat, 2.8g Fiber, 164.4 Calories

Roasted Asparagus Recipe

INGREDIENTS:

- ➢ 1 1/2 pounds Asparagus, 2 tablespoons Extra Virgin Olive Oil

- ➢ 1 teaspoon Salt & 1/2 teaspoon Black Pepper

DIRECTIONS:

- At first Heat oven to 400° & Line a jelly roll pan with aluminum foil.

- Next Rinse asparagus, and snap off tough ends. Lightly pat dry.

- Then Spread asparagus out in pan. Drizzle with olive oil and sprinkle with salt and pepper.

- After that Mix with your hands to distribute seasonings.

- Meanwhile Pat into a single layer.

- Later Bake until asparagus are tender and lightly crisped; about 15 minutes. Shake pan once or twice during baking time.

- Finally when the dish is ready to serve, serve it and enjoy!!!

Nutriotional Info:

3.8g Protein, 7g Fat , 3.6g Fiber, 94.4 Calories

Chicken and Okra Gumbo Recipe

Prep Time: 45 Minutes, Cook Time: 120 Minutes,
SERVINGS : 6, Points Value:11

INGREDIENTS:

- ➤ 1 tablespoon Olive Oil, 32 oz, with bone, cooked (yield after bone removed) Rotisserie Chicken & 6 cups (8 fluid ounces) Chicken Stock

- ➤ 1/2 cup Butter, 1/2 cup Whole Grain Soy Flour & 1 medium (2-1/2" diameter) Onions

- ➤ 1/2 medium (approx 2-3/4" long, 2-1/2" diameter) Bell Peppers, 1 stalk, medium (7-1/2" - 8" long) Celery & 3 cloves Garlic

- ➤ 1 1/4 each Bay Leaf, 1 tsp, ground Thyme (Dried)

- ➤ 1 teaspoon Oregano, 1/4 teaspoon Red or Cayenne Pepper & 16 ounces Okra

DIRECTIONS:

- At first Simplify this recipe by using the meat from a whole cooked rotisserri chicken. You will also need to have 6 cups of prepared chicken stock instead of using the water the chicken was cooked in.

- Next Everything may be cooked in the Dutch oven or crock pot.

- Then Cook for 1-2 hours on low. If using this substitute start with step 3 and using chicken stock in step 5.

- After that In a 5-quart Dutch oven or heavy soup pot, heat oil over medium-high heat.

- Meanwhile Add chicken pieces (if using this method you will need 2 lbs) in a single layer and cook until golden on both sides, about 10 minutes, turning once halfway through.

- In the meatime Remove from heat and transfer chicken pieces to a stockpot.

- Later Add 12 cups water to stockpot, and bring to a boil over high heat; reduce heat to medium-low, and simmer 30 minutes. Meanwhile, place Dutch oven over low heat.

- Melt butter, then whisk in soy flour to make the roux. Continue to whisk, scraping up any browned bits from the bottom of pan, until smooth, about 3 minutes.

- Cook the roux, whisking, until it reaches a deep caramel color, about 30 minutes.

- While roux cooks dice the onion, bell pepper and celery.

- After the roux has cooked for 30 minutes add the vegetables to the roux. Increase heat to medium and cook the vegetables, stirring often, until softened, about 5 minutes.

- Transfer chicken to a platter; let stand until cool enough to handle.

- Reserve the water the chicken cooked in.

- Stir garlic into roux mixture, and cook 2 minutes.

- Stir in bay leaves, thyme, oregano and cayenne. Cook 2 minutes more.

- Whisk 6 cups of the water the chicken cooked in into roux mixture (reserve or freeze remaining liquid for another use) and bring to a boil over medium-high heat.

- Add okra, return to a boil and cook 3 minutes.

- Reduce heat to low and keep at a simmer.

- Remove skin from chicken and separate meat from bones, discarding skin and bones.

- Shred meat into large pieces and add to Dutch oven; cover and cook 1 hour.

- Finally Season to taste with salt and pepper and serve.

Nutriotional Info:

33.9g Protein, 33.8g Fat, 4.3g Fiber, 487.1 Calories

Keto Chicken Liver Pate Recipe

Prep Time: 60 Minutes, Cook Time: 50 Minutes,
SERVINGS :6, Points Value: 3

INGREDIENTS:

- ➢ 1/2 pound Chicken Liver, 1/3 cup Chicken Broth, Bouillon or Consomme & 2 medium (4-1/8" long) Scallions or Spring Onions

- ➢ 1/8 teaspoon Allspice Ground, 1/4 cup Unsalted Butter Stick & 1/2 teaspoon Salt

- ➢ 1/4 teaspoon Black Pepper & 1/4 cup Heavy Cream

DIRECTIONS:

- At first In a small saucepan, combine chicken livers, broth, diced green onions and allspice.

- Next Bring to a boil; reduce heat and simmer 10 minutes until livers are cooked through.

- Then Drain and cool 20 minutes.

- After that Transfer mixture to a food processor, add butter, salt and black pepper, process until smooth. Transfer to a bowl, cover with plastic wrap and freeze 10 minutes.

- Meanwhile In a small bowl, beat the cream until stiff peaks form.

- In the meantime Fold cream into liver mixture.

- Later Transfer a serving bowl and cover with plastic wrap; refrigerate 1 hour until chilled.

- Finally Serve with toast points or low-carb crackers - remember to add in the additional carbs.

Nutriotional Info:

5.3g Protein, 9.9g Fat, 0.1g Fiber, 112.4 Calories

String Bean Salad Recipe

INGREDIENTS:

- ➤ 3/4 pound Green Snap Beans, 1 tablespoon Extra Virgin Olive Oil & 1/3 tablespoon Red Wine Vinegar

- ➤ 1/3 tablespoon chopped Shallots, 1 tablespoon Parsley

- ➤ 1/8 teaspoon Salt & 1/8 teaspoon Black Pepper

DIRECTIONS:

- At first Bring a medium saucepan of salted water fitted with a steamer basket to a boil.

- Next Add beans to basket and steam for 2 minutes.

- Then Drain, rinse beans in cold water and spread out on a dish towel to cool and dry.

- After that Mix together beans, oil, vinegar, shallot, parsley, salt and black pepper.

- Finally Serve at room temperature.

Nutriotional Info:

1.6g Protein, 3.5g Fat, 2.9g Fiber, 57.3 Calories

Atkins Chocolate Mint Cheesecake

Prep Time: 270 Minutes, Cook Time: 20 Minutes

Servings: 8, Points Value: 6

INGREDIENTS:

- ➢ 2 ounces Unsweetened Baking Chocolate Squares, 2 1/4 cups Heavy Cream & 1/4 cup Unsalted Butter Stick

- ➢ 1/2 cup Erythritol, 2 teaspoons Vanilla Extract & 2 large Eggs (Whole)

- ➢ 1 1/3 cups Tap Water, 1 3/4 cups Sucralose Based Sweetener (Sugar Substitute) & 1/4 cup Cocoa Powder (Unsweetened)

- ➢ 1 cup Blanched Almond Flour, 1 1/2 teaspoons Baking Powder (Straight Phosphate, Double Acting) & 1/2 teaspoon Salt

- ➢ 1 package (1 oz) Gelatin Powder (Unsweetened), 16 ounces Cream Cheese

- ➢ 1/8 tsp extract of Peppermint (Mint) & 8 tablespoons Hershey's Sugar Free Chocolate Syrup

DIRECTIONS:

- ▪ Be sure to use powdered erythritol (you will need about 1/2 cup granulated to make 1 cup powdered).

- ▪ It can be easily powdered in a blender. Measure it after it is powdered.

Bottom layer:

- At first Preheat an oven to 350°F and grease a 9x13x2-inch non-stick pan; set aside.

- Next Melt the chocolate and 1/4 cup heavy cream in a small bowl in the microwave at 20 second intervals. Once melted mix to combine and set aside to cool.

- Then Cream the butter and 1 cup powdered erythritol in a mixer for 5 minutes until light and fluffy.

- After that Add the vanilla and the eggs one at a time blending for 30 seconds between each egg.

- Meanwhile Add the cooled chocolate mixture, beating until thoroughly combined.

- After a while Add 1/3 cup water and 1/2 cup sucralose, beat for 1 minute.

- In the meantime In a small bowl whisk together the cocoa powder, almond flour, baking powder and salt. Add to the batter and mix for another minute until fully blended.

- Finally Pour batter into prepared pan and bake for 20 minutes or until a toothpick inserted in the center comes out clean. Allow to cool. While cooling prepare the top layer.

Top layer:

- Add the packet of gelatin to 1 cup boiling water.

- Mix until all the gelatin dissolves then place in the refrigerator about 10 minutes (do not allow it to fully set-up, cool to room temperature only.)

- In a medium bowl beat the softened cream cheese with 1 cup sucralose until fully blended and smooth.

- Add the peppermint extract and enough green food coloring to achieve desired color depth (about 1/4 teaspoon). When the gelatin has fully cooled, blend it into the cheese mixture.

- Whip the remaining 2 cups cream with the remaining 1/4 cup sucralose until semi-stiff peaks form.

- Gently fold the cream into the cheese mixture until fully incorporated.

- Pour this over the cooled brownie layer in the pan and refrigerate for 4 hours or overnight.

- When ready to serve, cut into 24 squares and top with 1 teaspoon of sugar-free chocolate syrup (Smucker's Sugar Free Sundae Syrup works great as it is a little thicker than regular syrup.)

- To make spider web: starting in the middle of the square make a spiral. Take a toothpick and from the center pull out in a straight line to the outer edge. Repeat 5-6 times spacing them equally

- Finally when the dish is ready to serve, serve it and enjoy!!!!

Nutriotional Info:

4.9g Protein, 20.8g Fat, 1.1g Fiber, 219.8 Calories

Spring Vegetable Soup Recipe

Prep Time: 10 Minutes, Cook Time: 15 Minutes,
SERVINGS : 8, Points Value: 2

INGREDIENTS:

- ➢ 3 tablespoons Vegetable Oil, 4 each Leeks & 1/2 pound Asparagus

- ➢ 1 large Summer Squash, 4 ounces Snowpeas (Pea Pod) & 1/2 teaspoon Salt

- ➢ 1/4 teaspoon Black Pepper, 3 14.5 ounces cans Chicken Broth, Bouillon or Consomme

- ➢ 14 1/2 fluid ounces Tap Water, 1/4 cup Parsley & 1 teaspoon Lemon Peel

DIRECTIONS:

- ▪ At first Heat oil in a large soup pot over medium-high heat.

- ▪ Next Add leeks and cook 2 minutes, until softened, stirring occasionally.

- ▪ Then Add asparagus and cook 2 minutes, until color brightens.

- ▪ After that Add squash and pea pods and cook 2 minutes, or until squash begins to soften. Add salt, pepper, broth and water; bring to a boil.

- ▪ Meanwhile Reduce heat to low and simmer 5 minutes, until vegetables are tender.

- ▪ Finally Just before serving, stir in parsley and lemon zest.

Nutriotinal Info:

5.5g Protein, 6.3g Fat, 2.3g Fiber, 117.4 Calories

Keto Fruit-Glazed Pork Over Mixed Greens Recipe

Prep Time: 10 Minutes, Cook Time: 40 Minutes,
SERVINGS : 5, Points Value: 10

INGREDIENTS:

- ➢ 3 pounds Pork Loin (Tenderloin), 1 3/4 teaspoons Salt & 1 teaspoon Black Pepper

- ➢ 5 tablespoons Extra Virgin Olive Oil, 5 1/3 tablespoons Sugar Free Orange Marmalade & 5 1/3 tablespoons Sugar Free Apricot Preserves

- ➢ 1/2 teaspoon Cinnamon, 1/2 tablespoon Balsamic Vinegar & 6 cups Spring Mix Salad

DIRECTIONS:

- At first Preheat oven to 400°F.

- Next Season tenderloins with 1 1/4 teaspoon salt and 1/2 teaspoon pepper.

- Then In a large skillet over medium-high high, heat 3 tablespoons of the oil. Brown pork for about 15 minutes, turning as needed.

- After that Transfer to a rimmed baking sheet lined with aluminum foil and place in oven. Roast pork for 15 minutes.

- Meanwhile, in a small bowl whisk together orange marmalade, apricot jam and cinnamon.

- Transfer 1 tablespoon of the jam mixture to a large bowl and set aside.

- After the pork has roasted for 20 minutes, brush pork generously with jam mixture, allowing any excess to drip onto the pan.

- Meanwhile Turn oven up to 450°F and roast for another 5 minutes more or until just cooked through and a meat thermometer registers 160°F.

- Later Transfer to a cutting board and let pork stand for 5 minutes before cutting into 1-inch slices on the bias.

- In the meantime To make the dressing, mix the reserved jam mixture with the vinegar, and remaining salt and pepper.

- Slowly whisk in the remaining oil. Add greens and toss to coat.

- Divide greens on 6 plates and top with pork slices and any accumulated juices and jam from the pan.

- Finally when the dish is ready to serve, serve it and enjoy!!!!

Nutritional Info:

47.3g Protein, 23.5g Fat, 4.4g Fiber, 435 Calories

Keto Chicken Legs Amandine Recipe

Prep Time: 10 Minutes, Cook Time: 30 Minutes,
SERVINGS : 6, Points Value: 14

INGREDIENTS:

- ➤ 2 tablespoons Canola Vegetable Oil, 24 ounces Chicken Leg, bone-in, with skin & 1/4 cup sliced Almonds

- ➤ 4 fluid ounces Sauvignon Blanc Wine & 1/4 cup Tap Water

- ➤ 1 1/2 teaspoons Garlic, 2 tablespoons Unsalted Butter Stick

- ➤ 2 tablespoons Parsley & 1 tablespoon Fresh Lemon Juice

DIRECTIONS:

- At first Heat oven to warm setting. Heat oil in a large nonstick skillet over high heat.

- Next Sprinkle chicken legs with salt and pepper.

- Then Brown chicken 3 to 4 minutes on each side.

- After that Reduce heat to low, cover and cook 30 minutes, until chicken is cooked through. Transfer to a platter and place in oven.

- Meanwhile Add almonds to skillet; cook 2 to 3 minutes, until golden.

- Moreover Transfer to a plate with a slotted spoon.

- In the meantime Pour off fat from skillet. Add wine, water and minced garlic to skillet. Increase heat to high and cook, stirring occasionally, until mixture is reduced by half.

- Later Remove from heat and stir in almonds, butter, parsley and lemon juice.

- Spoon sauce over chicken.

- Finally when the dish is ready to serve, serve it and enjoy!!!

Nutrional Info:

45.6g Protein, 38.6g Fat, 0.8g Fiber, 567.9 Calories

Low Carb Cajun Shrimp and Sausage Skillet

Prep Time: 15 Minutes, Cook Time: 20 Minutes,

4 SERVINGS , Points Value: 9

INGREDIENTS:

- ➢ 14 ounces smoked cajun style andouille pork sausage, 2 tablespoons butter, unsalted & 16 ounces raw shrimp, large

- ➢ 2 tablespoons cajun seasoning, 1/3 cup fresh white onion, chopped & 3/4 cup fresh red bell pepper

- ➢ 1 teaspoon fresh garlic, 1 teaspoon fresh rosemary & 1/3 cup sauvignon blanc white wine, table

- ➢ 1 1/2 cups chicken broth & 1 1/2 tablespoons canned tomato paste, 6 oz, unsalted

- ➢ 1 teaspoon lime juice, 100%, fresh squeezed, 1 ea fresh avocado & 1 tablespoon fresh chives

DIRECTIONS:

- ▪ At first In a large skillet over medium heat, brown ½-inch slices of sausage, 3-4 minutes per side.

- ▪ Next Scrape into a medium bowl and set aside.

- ▪ Then Thaw and rinse shrimp, then dry on a paper towel lined plate & Sprinkle shrimp with 1 ½ tablespoons Cajun seasoning.

- ▪ After that In the large skillet over medium heat, melt 1 tablespoon butter.

- ▪ Meanwhile Add seasoned shrimp in a single layer and cook until opaque and cooked through, 4-5 minutes, flipping once mid-way through.

- In the meantime Scrape into the bowl with the sausage.

- Moreover Melt remaining butter in the skillet over medium heat.

- After a while Add onion and sauté, stirring frequently, until becoming translucent, 3 minutes.

- Later Add garlic and sauté until fragrant, 30 seconds.

- At one point Add red bell pepper and sauté for another 3 minutes to soften.

- Gradually Sprinkle vegetables with rosemary and remaining ½ tablespoon Cajun seasoning, sautéing until fragrant, another 30 seconds.

- Pour white wine in, stirring and allow to simmer until reduced, about 2 minutes. Pour in chicken broth, whisk in tomato paste, and simmer until well combined and slightly thickened.

- Add shrimp and sausage back in and simmer until heated through.

- Finally Before serving, drizzle with lime juice, mix in cubed avocado, and garnish with chopped fresh chives. One serving is about 1 ½ cups shrimp and sausage with veggies and sauce.

Nutriotional Info:

32.1g Protein, 26.1g Fat, 4.9g Fiber, 494.8 Calories

Spicy Maple Chicken Wings Recipe

Prep Time: 10 Minutes, Cook Time: 45 Minutes,
SERVINGS : 6, Points Value: 4

INGREDIENTS:

- ➤ 8 ounces Crushed Tomatoes (Canned) & 1 cup (8 fluid ounces) Water

- ➤ 1/2 cup Sugar Free Maple Flavored Syrup, 2 tablespoons Poultry Seasoning 7 1 1/2 teaspoons Garlic

- ➤ 32 oz, with bone, raw (yield after cooking, bone removed) Chicken Wing

DIRECTIONS:

- In a large saucepot over high heat, bring tomato purée, water, syrup, chicken seasoning and garlic to a boil.

- Separate the wings at the joint and discard the wing tips.

- Add wings to pot, turn heat down to low, cover and simmer 5 minutes.

- Uncover and cook 20 minutes more until wings are cooked through.

- Transfer wings to a platter and continue cooking until liquid thickens to form a glaze, about 10 more minutes.

- Season to taste with hot sauce (Tobasco, if desired), salt and pepper.

- Add chicken wings back to pot and toss to coat well.

- Heat broiler; arrange wings on broiler pan.

- Broil until crisp, about 5 minutes per side.

- Finally when the dish is ready to serve, serve it and enjoy!!!!

Nutriotional Info:

15g Protein, 10.5g Fat, 6.5g Fiber, 187.2 Calories

Swedish Red Cabbage Recipe

Prep Time: 10 Minutes, Cook Time: 35 Minutes,
SERVINGS :8, Points Value: 1

INGREDIENTS:

- ➢ 1/4 cup Unsalted Butter Stick & 2 medium (2-3/4" diameter) (approx 3 per pound) Apples

- ➢ 2 pounds Cabbage, 1 teaspoon Salt & 1 tablespoon Sucralose Based Sweetener (Sugar Substitute)

- ➢ 2 tablespoons Vinegar (Cider) & 1/4 teaspoon Allspice Ground

- ➢ 1 small Red Onion & 2 2/3 fluid ounces Red Table Wine

DIRECTIONS:

- At first Shred cabbag & Melt butter in a large, heavy Dutch oven over medium-high heat.

- Next Add chopped apples and onion. Cook 10 minutes, stirring occasionally, until tender.

- Then Stir in cabbage and cook 8 minutes more, stirring frequently, until slightly wilted.

- After that Stir in sugar substitute, vinegar, salt and allspice.

- Meanwhile Cover and cook 10 minutes, stirring occasionally. Uncover, add wine.

- Later Cook 10-15 minutes more, until very tender.

- Finally Season to taste with salt and pepper & serve.

Nutrional Info:

1.9g Protein, 6g Fat, 3.6g Fiber, 109.5 Calories

Mixed Vegetable Kebabs Recipe

Prep Time: 30 Minutes, Cook Time: 20 Minutes,
SERVINGS : 6, Points Value: 2

INGREDIENTS:

> 1 eggplant, peeled (yield from 1-1/4 lb) Eggplant & 1 large (2-1/4 per pound, approx 3-3/4" long, 3" diameter) Sweet Red Peppers

> 1 pepper, large (3-3/4" long, 3" dia) Yellow Sweet Peppers, 1 medium Zucchini & 1 medium Yellow Summer Squash

> 12 Cherry Tomatoes, 1 1/4 teaspoons Salt & 1/4 teaspoon Black Pepper

> 3 tablespoons Extra Virgin Olive Oil, 1 tablespoon chopped Shallots & 2 tablespoons Red Wine Vinegar

> 11 1/2 leaves Basil & 1/2 ounce Basil

DIRECTIONS:

▪ You will need six 12-inch bamboo skewers, soaked for 20 minutes in warm water before skewering the vegetables.

For the kebabs:

▪ At first Spread eggplant cubes in a single layer on a baking sheet lined with paper towels; sprinkle with 3/4 teaspoon of the salt, and let stand 15 minutes. Pat dry.

▪ Next Heat grill to medium-low.

▪ Then Cube all remaining vegetables, leave the tomatoes whole and place in a large bowl.

- After that Toss vegetables with the remaining 1/2 teaspoon salt and the pepper.

- Let sit 1 minute, then combine with the eggplant and 1 Tbsp oil tossing until well coated.

- Meanwhile Thread each skewer with 2 pieces each of red and yellow bell pepper, 2 pieces squash or zucchini, 2 cubes eggplant and 2 cherry tomatoes wrapped in basil leaves.

- Cover with plastic wrap until grill is ready.

- In the meantime Grill kebabs until vegetables are softened and lightly browned, 15 to 20 minutes, turning every 5 minutes.

For the dressing:

- At first In a small bowl, whisk the remaining 2 tablespoons oil, chopped shallots, vinegar and chopped basil until well combined.

- Next Cover, and set aside.

- Once cooked, arrange kebabs on a serving platter, and drizzle with dressing.

- Finally Serve immediately.

Nutriotional Info:

2.6 gm protein, 7.3 gm fat, 4.7 gm fiber, 112.4 gm calories

Chicken Salad Sandwich with Grapes and Walnuts Recipe

Prep Time: 20 Minutes, Cook Time: 0 Minutes, SERVINGS: 4, Points Value: 12

INGREDIENTS:

- ➢ 1/2 cup chopped English Walnuts, 24 ounce raw (yield after cooking, bone removed) Chicken Breast & 1/2 cup Real Mayonnaise

- ➢ 1/2 cup, seedles Grapes (Red or Green, European Type Varieties Such As Thompson Seedless) & 1/2 cup chopped Red Onions

- ➢ 1/4 cup chopped Celery , 1 dash Salt

- ➢ 1 dash Black Pepper & 2 servings Mama Lupes Low Carb Tortillas

DIRECTIONS:

- ▪ At first Heat oven to 400°F.

- ▪ Next Spread walnuts in a single layer on a baking sheet and toast until fragrant and golden brown, about 5 minutes.

- ▪ Then Place chicken in a medium saucepan and cover with cold water.

- ▪ After that Bring to a simmer and poach chicken is cooked through but still tender, about 12 minutes.

- ▪ Meanwhile Remove from saucepan and cool slightly.

- ▪ In the meantime Cut warm chicken into ½-inch chunks and place in a mixing bowl.

- ▪ Later Add mayonnaise, walnuts, grapes, onion and celery and mix well. Season with salt and pepper.

- Finally Stuff chicken salad into pita pocket halves and serve, or chill until ready to eat.

Nutriotional Info:

31.7g Protein, 38g Fat, 3.5g Fiber, 504.3 Calories

Keto Buffalo Chicken Egg Salad Recipe

INGREDIENTS:

➢ 6 large Boiled Eggs, 6 ounces boneless, cooked Chicken Thigh & 3 tablespoons Real Mayonnaise

➢ 1 1/2 tablespoons Red Hot Buffalo Wing Sauce

➢ 1/4 cup, crumbled Blue or Roquefort Cheese & 8 stalk, medium (7-1/2" - 8" long) Celery

DIRECTIONS:

- At first Be sure to use a Buffalo hot sauce that has only a few ingredients including red pepper, vinegar and salt; 0g NC per serving.

- Next Also pre-cooked rotisseri chicken can be used instead of cooking the chicken.

- Hard boil the eggs: Then cover 6 eggs with water, bring to a boil, remove from heat and allow to sit for 10 minutes.

- Immediately plunge eggs into an ice water bath, allow to cool then peel and dice. Reserve in a medium bowl.

- While eggs are cooking if your chicken is raw, cook chicken over medium heat in a skillet or on the grill until the juices run clear and the meat is no longer pink in the center.

- Let it Cool and dice; add to the eggs in the bowl.

- To the bowl with the diced eggs and chicken add the mayonnaise, Buffalo hot sauce and blue cheese.

- Moreover Mix to combine and blend flavors.

- Later Add salt and pepper to taste. Serve with celery stalks for dipping or carefully fill celery stalks.

- Finally Drizzle with additional Buffalo hot sauce as a garnish or if more heat is desired.

Nutriotional Info:

11.2g Protein, 12.3g Fat, 0.6g Fiber, 164.1 Calories

Southwest Garden Salad Recipe

Prep Time: 20 Minutes, Cook Time: 0 Minutes

SERVINGS : 4, Points Value: 14

INGREDIENTS:

- ➢ 1 fruit (2" diameter) Lime, 1 cup Cilantro (Coriander) , 1/2 teaspoon Cumin & 1/2 teaspoon Salt

- ➢ 1/2 cup Extra Virgin Olive Oil, 2 cups shredded Monterey Jack Cheese & 8 cups shredded Cos or Romaine Lettuce

- ➢ 1 cup slice Cucumber (with Peel), 1/2 pepper, large (3-3/4" long, 3" dia) Yellow Sweet Peppers & 1/8 teaspoon Black Pepper

- ➢ 1 fruit without skin and seed California Avocado & 1 cup cherry tomato Red Tomato

DIRECTIONS:

Make dressing:

- ▪ At firstJuice and zest the lime.

- ▪ Next Place cilantro, lime juice, lime zest, cumin and half of salt in a blender.

- ▪ Then Turn on motor and drizzle in oil in a slow, steady stream.

- ▪ After that Toss lettuce, 1 cup of cheese, cucumber and yellow pepper with dressing.

- ▪ Meanwhile Season with black pepper and remaining salt and mound on 4 plates.

- ▪ Finally To serve, top with avocado, halved tomatoes and remaining cheese.

Nutriotional Info:

16.8g Protein, 51.3g Fat, 6.3g Fiber ,561.6 Calories

Keto Beef Tenderloin Recipe

Prep Time: 20 Minutes, Cook Time: 30 Minutes,
SERVINGS : 5, Points Value: 18

INGREDIENTS:

- ➤ 4 pounds Beef Tenderloin (Trimmed to 1/4" Fat, Prime Grade) & 1 1/2 tablespoons Extra Virgin Olive Oil

- ➤ 1 teaspoon Salt & 1/2 teaspoon Black Pepper

DIRECTIONS:

- At first Heat oven to 425°F.

- Next Place beef in a jelly-roll pan.

- Then Rub with oil, salt and pepper. Insert a meat thermometer.

- After that Roast 30 to 35 minutes for medium-rare doneness.

- Meanwhile Thermometer should register 125°F.

- Later Transfer to a cutting board; loosely tent with foil and let rest 10 minutes before slicing.

- Finally when the dish is ready to serve, serve it and enjoy!!!

Nutriotional Info:

40.6g Protein, 54.8g Fat , 0g Fiber, 666.8 Calories

Grilled Chicken Breast with Avocado, Cheese and Tomato Salad Recipe

Prep Time: 10 Minutes, Cook Time: 10 Minutes

SERVING : 4, Points Value: 17

INGREDIENTS:

- ➢ 1 serving Keto Italian Dressing, 1 breast, bone and skin removed Skinless Chicken Breast & 2 cup, shredded or choppeds Mixed Salad Greens

- ➢ 3 each Cherry or Grape Tomato, 1/2 fruit without skin and seed California Avocados & 1 ounce Monterey Jack Cheese

DIRECTIONS:

- At first Use the Atkins recipe to make Italian Dressing for the salad, you will need 2 tablespoons.

- Next Preheat a grill. Season chicken with salt and freshly ground black pepper.

- Then Grill over medium heat until the juices run clear and it is no longer pink in the center, about 5 minutes per side depending upon the thickness.

- While the chicken is cooking, combine the greens, halved tomatoes, sliced avocado and shredded cheese with the dressing.

- Finally Toss to combine and serve immediately with the chicken.

Nutriotional Info:

65.4g Protein, 45.5g Fat, 8.9g Fiber, 720.1 Calories

Spaghetti Squash Salad Recipe

Prep Time: 135 Minutes, Cook Time: 45 Minutes,
SERVINGS : 6, Points Value:

INGREDIENTS:

- ➢ 5 cups Cooked Spaghetti Squash, 1/4 cup Extra Virgin Olive Oil & 4 medium (4-1/8" long) Scallions or Spring Onions

- ➢ 1/4 cup Parsley, 1/4 cup Cilantro (Coriander)

- ➢ 1/2 teaspoon Salt & 1/4 teaspoon Black Pepper

DIRECTIONS:

- Before beginning this recipe, prepare spaghetti squash.

- Next You will need about a 2-2.5 lb squash.

- Then Prick the squash in several places and bake 45 minutes until tender in a preheated 400°F oven.

- After that Allow to cool slightly; cut in half, lengthwise; and scoop out seeds and discard. Pull out squash strands from each side with a fork.

- Meanwhile Transfer to a bowl to cool.

- Alternatively, cut the squash in half, remove the seeds, place cut-side down on a microwaves safe plate and heat on high heat for 5 minutes at a time checking in between heatings to see when it has fully cooked through (about 10-15 minutes).

- In the meantime Whisk the olive oil with the green onions, parsley, cilantro, salt, and pepper. Pour over baked, cooled squash; toss until well combined.

- Refrigerate 2 hours for flavors to blend.

- Finally when the dish is ready to serve, serve it and enjoy!!!

Nutriotional Info:

1.1g Protein, 12.5g Fat, 2.3g Fiber, 146.7 Calories

Keto Apricot-Glazed Brisket Recipe

Prep Time: 10 Minutes, Cook Time: 210 Minutes,
SERVINGS : 5, Points Value: 9

INGREDIENTS:

- ➢ 4 pounds Beef Brisket (Whole, Lean Only), 2 teaspoons Salt & 2 teaspoons Paprika

- ➢ 1 teaspoon Black Pepper, 3 tablespoons Sugar Free Apricot Preserves

- ➢ 1 large Onions, raw & 3 medium Carrots, raws

DIRECTIONS:

- At first Heat oven to 475°F. Season brisket with salt, paprika and pepper.

- Next Place brisket fat side down in a Dutch oven.

- Then Scatter quartered onions and diced carrots around the beef. Cook 15 minutes.

- After that Turn brisket fat side up and add 1/2 cup water.

- Meanwhile Cover tightly & Reduce oven temperature to 300°F.

- In the meantime Cook 3 to 4 hours, until tender and an instant-read meat thermometer inserted in center registers 180°F.

- Later Heat broiler & Remove brisket from Dutch oven and place on a broiler pan.

- Moreover Spread jam over brisket & Broil 6 from heat source 5 minutes, until jam is lightly browned in spots.

- While brisket is broiling, remove onions and carrots from cooking juices.

- Cover brisket with foil and allow to rest 15 minutes before serving.

- Finally Remove surface fat with a spoon and serve with degreased cooking juices.

- The carrots and onions will be very soft but if purreed in a blender make a nice side dish with the beef.

Nutritional Info:

47.5g Protein, 16.9g Fat, 2g Fiber, 374 Calories

Beef and Vegetable Stew Recipe

Prep Time: 10 Minutes, Cook Time: 165 Minutes,
SERVINGS :5, Points Value: 5

INGREDIENTS:

- ➢ 2 tablespoons Extra Virgin Olive Oil, 1 1/2 pounds Beef Chuck (Mock Tender Steak, Lean Only, Trimmed to 1/4" Fat) & 1 teaspoon leaf Dried Thyme Leaves

- ➢ 1 teaspoon leaf Oregano, 1 teaspoon Rosemary (Dried) & 1 teaspoon Paprika

- ➢ 2 teaspoons Salt, 1 teaspoon Black Pepper & 2 tablespoons Unsalted Butter Stick

- ➢ 1 cup White Pearl Onions, 2 cloves Garlic & 16 fluid ounces Merlot Wine

- ➢ 1 pound Green Snap Beans, 1 medium Carrot & 2 teaspoons Dixie Diners' Thick It Up

DIRECTIONS:

- ▪ At first Heat oven to 325°F & Heat half the oil in a Dutch oven over medium-high heat.

- ▪ Next Toss beef with thyme, oregano, rosemary, paprika, salt and pepper.

- ▪ Then Brown half the beef; transfer to a bowl. Repeat with remaining oil and beef.

- ▪ After that Set asid & Melt butter in Dutch oven or crock pot.

- ▪ Meanwhile Add diced onions; cook 7 - 8 minutes until onions begin to brown.

- ▪ In the meantime Add minced garlic during last 2 minutes of cooking time.

- After a while Add reserved meat and accumulated juices, wine and 2 cups water.

- In the next step Bring to a boil & Cover Dutch oven and place in oven.

- Moreover Cook 2 hours, until beef is tender.

- Add green beans and carrots; cook 15 minutes more, just until beans and carrots are tender & Transfer Dutch oven to stove top over medium-high heat.

- Stir in thickener; cook 2 minutes more, stirring, until sauce thickens.

- Finally Adjust seasonings to taste and serve immediately.

Nutritional Info:

23.3g Protein, 12.4g Fat, 4.2g Fiber, 305 Calories

Open-Sesame Broccoli Salad Recipe

Prep Time: 30 Minutes, Cook Time: 10 Minutes,
SERVINGS : 6, Points Value: 1

INGREDIENTS:

➤ 8 cup flowerets Broccoli Flower Clusters, 2 tablespoons Dried Whole Sesame Seeds & 2 tablespoons Tamari Soybean Sauce

➤ 2 tablespoons Sodium and Sugar Free Rice Vinegar, 2 teaspoons Toasted Sesame Oil & 2 teaspoons Sucralose Based Sweetener (Sugar Substitute)

DIRECTIONS:

- Factor in half an hour to marinate this salad to allow the flavors to blend. Or prepare ahead of time and refrigerate for up to 24 hours.

- This recipe is suitable for all phases of the Atkins diet except for the first two weeks of Induction due to the sesame seeds.

- At first In a large pot fitted with a steamer basket, bring water to a boil and steam broccoli 5 minutes until crisp-tender.

- Next Rinse under cold water; drain.

- Then In dry skillet over medium heat, toast sesame seeds 5 minutes, until golden and fragrant, stirring frequently to prevent burning. Transfer to small plate to cool.

- After that In large bowl, combine tamari, vinegar, oil and sugar substitute and mix well.

- Meanwhile Add broccoli and half the sesame seeds and toss well.

- Later Marinate at room temperature at least 30 minutes, stirring occasionally.

- Finally Before serving, sprinkle broccoli with remaining sesame seeds.

Nutriotional Info:

3g Protein, 2.5g Fat, 0.3g Fiber, 46.9 Calories

Keto Chili Bowl Recipe

Prep Time: 15 Minutes, Cook Time: 20 Minutes,
SERVINGS : 5, Points Value: 10

INGREDIENTS:

- ➢ 1 tablespoon Extra Virgin Olive Oil, 1 medium (2-1/2" diameter) Onions & 2 each Garlic, clove

- ➢ 2 Jalapeno Peppers, 2 tablespoons Chili Powder & 1 1/2 teaspoons Cumin

- ➢ 1/2 teaspoon Salt, 1/4 teaspoon Red or Cayenne Pepper & 1/4 teaspoon Black Pepper, ground

- ➢ 1/8 teaspoon Cinnamon, 2 pounds Ground Beef (80% Lean / 20% Fat)

- ➢ 1 14.5 ounces can Diced Tomato, 1 1/2 cups shredded Monterey Jack Cheese

DIRECTIONS:

- At first Heat broiler. In a deep 9 or 10-inch oven-proof skillet, heat olive oil over medium-high heat for 1 minute.

- Next Add chopped onion; cook until golden, about 3 minutes, stirring occasionally and reducing heat to medium if needed to prevent scorching.

- Then Add minced or pressed garlic and diced jalapeños; cook 30 seconds, stirring until fragrant.

- After that Add chili powder, cumin, salt, red pepper, black pepper, and cinnamon; stir to coat the vegetables.

- Meanwhile Add ground beef and cook until browned, about 6-10 minutes, stirring occasionally.

- Later Drain excess liquid from pan.

- Moreover Add tomatoes, and bring to a boil. Sprinkle cheese over top.

- After a while Place 5 inches from heating element, and broil just until melted, 2-3 minutes.

- One serving is about 3/4 cup of chili.

- Finally when the dish is ready to serve , serve it and enjoy!!!!

Nutriotional Info:

25.6g Protein, 31.2g Fat, 1.5g Fiber, 411.3 Calories

Keto Bahian Halibut Recipe

INGREDIENTS:

- ➢ 2 tablespoons Extra Virgin Olive Oil, 2 tablespoons Fresh Lime Juice & 2 pounds Atlantic and Pacific Halibut

- ➢ 4 tablespoons chopped Onions, 1 cup chopped Green Sweet Pepper & 1 pepper Serrano Pepper

- ➢ 1 teaspoon Garlic , 1 teaspoon Salt

- ➢ 1/2 cup Coconut Cream & 1 small whole (2-2/5" diameter) Red Tomato

DIRECTIONS:

- At first With a fork, whisk 1 tablespoon oil and all the lime juice on large platter, add fish, and turn to coat.

- Next Dice the onion, bell pepper and the serrano pepper (be sure to use gloves to protect your hands from the heat of the pepper - do not include the seeds or ribs if you want to reduce the heat).

- Then Mince the garlic and add to a bowl with the onions and peppers.

- After that Chop the tomatoes, place in a small bowl and set aside.

- Meanwhile Heat remaining tablespoon oil in a 12-inch nonstick skillet over medium heat.

- In the meantime Add garlic and the diced onion and peppers.

- After a while Cook 6 minutes until onion is translucent and peppers are just tender.

- Gradually Sprinkle 1/2 teaspoon of salt over fish and add fish to skillet; pour coconut milk over fish and add tomato.

- Moreover Reduce heat to medium-low and simmer 8 to 9 minutes, turning fish halfway through cooking time.

- Finally Stir remaining salt into sauce, spoon over fish a few times, and serve immediately.

Nutriotional Info:

48.7g Protein, 18.6g Fat, 1.1g Fiber, 391.4 Calories

Red, White and Blue Coleslaw Recipe

INGREDIENTS:

- ➤ 3/4 cup(s) Mayonnaise (Bestfoods), 1/4 cup Sour Cream (Cultured)

- ➤ 1 cup, crumbled Blue or Roquefort Cheese , 1 1/3 tablespoons Red Wine Vinegar & 1/2 teaspoon Garlic

- ➤ 1 1/2 teaspoons Salt, 1/4 teaspoon Sucralose Based Sweetener (Sugar Substitute)

- ➤ 6 cups Red Cabbage, raw, shredded & 6 cups Green or White Cabbage, raw, shredded

DIRECTIONS:

- ▪ At first Combine mayonnaise, sour cream, blue cheese, vinegar, minced garlic, salt, and sugar substitute in a large bowl.

- ▪ Next Add green and red cabbage and toss well.

- ▪ Then Cover and chill at least 1 hour before serving.

- ▪ Can be made ahead.

- ▪ Later Store in an airtight container and refrigerate up to 24 hours.

- ▪ Finally when the dish is ready to serve, serve it and enjoy!!!!

Nutritional Info:

3.5g Protein, 15.2g Fat, 1.6g Fiber, 167.8Calories

Shortcut Moussaka Recipe

INGREDIENTS:

- ➢ 3 tablespoons Light Olive Oil, 1/2 small Onion & 2 teaspoons Garlic

- ➢ 24 ounces Ground Lamb, 1 tablespoon Tomato Paste & 4 fluid ounces Red Table Wine

- ➢ 1 cup Tomato Sauce, 1/2 teaspoon Salt & 1/4 teaspoon Cinnamon

- ➢ 1/8 teaspoon Cloves (Ground), 1 eggplant, peeled (yield from 1-1/4 lb) Eggplant

- ➢ 6 ounces Cream Cheese, 1/4 cup Heavy Cream

- ➢ 1/4 teaspoon Nutmeg (Ground) & 1/4 cup, crumbled Feta Cheese

DIRECTIONS:

- ▪ At first Preheat oven to 425° F & Heat 1 tablespoon oil in a large pan over medium-high heat.

- ▪ Next Sauté diced white onion until soft, about 3 minutes.

- ▪ Then Add minced garlic and sauté until aroma is released, about 30 seconds.

- ▪ Meanwhile Add lamb and sauté until still slightly pink, breaking up with a wooden spoon, about 4 minutes.

- After a while Drain off most of the fat, add tomato paste and sauté until lamb is cooked, about 1 minutes longer.

- In the next step Stir in wine, tomato sauce, salt, cinnamon and cloves.

- Later Bring to a boil; reduce heat to low and simmer 10 minutes to reduce sauce.

- While sauce is cooking, cut eggplant into slices and brush with remaining oil.

- Arrange in a single layer on a baking sheet and bake until lightly browned and slightly softened, about 12 minutes, turning once during cooking time.

- In a small saucepan whisk cream cheese, cream and nutmeg over medium heat and cook until cream cheese melts and mixture is smooth, about 3 minutes. Set aside.

- Turn oven down to 350°F.

- Spread a thin layer of meat sauce on bottom of an 8-inch square baking pan.

- Layer half the eggplant slices on top; cover with half the remaining meat sauce and half the cream sauce. Repeat layers.

- Sprinkle the top with feta cheese.

- Bake until cheese starts to brown, about 25 minutes.

- Finally Serve hot or at room temperature.

Nutriotional Info:

23.6g Protein, 48.7g, Fat, 3.5g Fiber, 586.4 Calories

Almond Muffin in a Minute Recipe

INGREDIENTS

➤ 1/4 cup Bob's Red Mill Almond Meal/Flour (1/4 cup is 28g) & 1 teaspoon No Calorie Sweetener

➤ 1/4 teaspoon Baking Powder (Straight Phosphate, Double Acting) & 1 dash Salt

➤ 1/2 teaspoon Cinnamon, 1 large Egg (Whole) & 1 teaspoon Canola Vegetable Oil

DIRECTIONS:

• At first Place all dry ingredients in a coffee mug. Stir to combine.

• Next Add the egg and oil. Stir until thoroughly combined.

• Then Microwave for 1 minute.

• LaterUse a knife if necessary to help remove the muffin from the cup, slice, butter, eat.

• Finally when the dish is ready to serve, serve it and enjoy!!!!

Nutriotional Info:

12.3g Protein, 23.5g Fat, 3.6g Fiber, 276.9 Calories

Keto Turkey and Mushroom Chowder Recipe

INGREDIENTS:

- ➤ 16 ounces Turkey Breast Meat (Fryer-Roasters, Cooked, Roasted) & 4 cups Chicken Broth, Bouillon or Consomme

- ➤ 3 cups Tap Water, 12 ounces Mushroom Pieces and Stems , 1 small Onion & 2 stalk, medium (7-1/2" - 8" long) Celery

- ➤ 1/2 teaspoon Garlic, 1/2 cup Pearled Barley (Cooked) & 3/4 cup Heavy Cream

DIRECTIONS

- ▪ At first In a soup pot, combine turkey bones (if available from leftover turkey), broth and water.

- ▪ Next Bring to a boil, lower heat and simmer for 30 minutes.

- ▪ Then Strain, discard bones and return broth to the pot.

- ▪ After that Bring broth back to a boil and add mushrooms, white onion, celery, garlic and barley.

- ▪ Meanwhile Adjust heat and simmer for 20 minutes.

- ▪ After a while Transfer 2 cups of the soup to a blender.

- ▪ Later Holding down the lid tightly, blend until smooth. Return to the pot.

- Moreover Stir in turkey meat and cream and cook until just heated through.

- Finally Garnish with parsley, and add salt and freshly ground pepper to taste and serve.

Nutriotional Info:

21.6g Protein, 9.6g Fat ,1.1g Fiber, 199 Calories

Made in the USA
Las Vegas, NV
20 September 2024

95533129R00046